The Superfood Power Smoothie Book

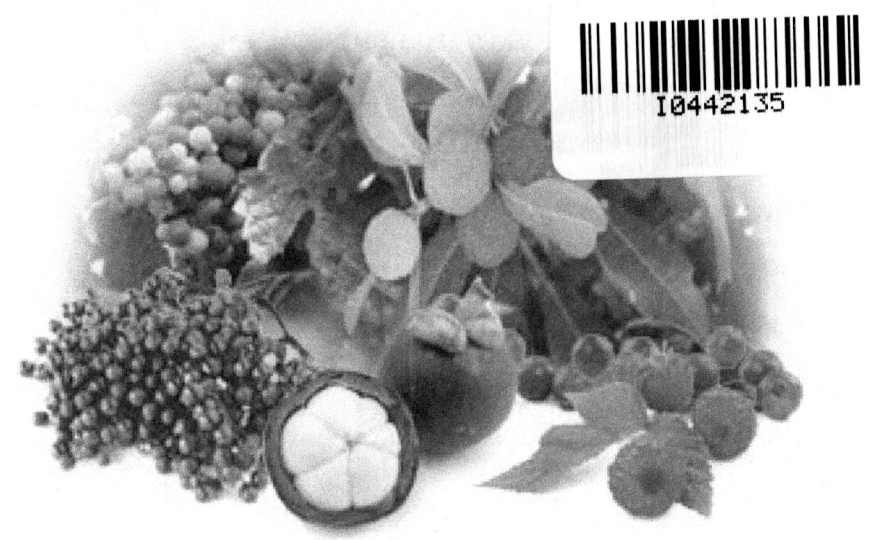

I0442135

Easy to Prepare Smoothie Recipes to Boost Your Health and Help You Lose Weight

By Melinda Rolf

Contents

Introduction 3

What's the Deal with Superfoods? 4

Discover these Impressive Nutritional Perks................5

What are Power/Superfood Ingredients?.....................7

What is the Special Ingredient of Superfoods? 8

Clearing Up a Misconception 9

The Exotic vs. the Ordinary 10

Why Choose Power/Superfood Smoothies? 11

More Reasons to Try Superfoods....................................12

What Ingredients are the Best to Make Superfood Smoothies? ...14

Avocadoes 15

Blueberries 15

Beans 15

Broccoli 16

Garlic..16

Dark Chocolate 16

Kiwi Fruit 17

Honey...18

Goji Berry (Sometimes spelled as Gogi berry).............18

Acai Berries...19

Cacao 20

Maca 20

Spirulina 20

Blue-Green Algae 21

Aloe 21

Power Smoothie Recipes to Boost Your Health...............22

Citrus Aloe Vera Smoothie Recipe 22

Coconut + Cranberry Power Smoothie 25

Pistachio Superfood Smoothie 26

The Energizer Smoothie 27

Spirulina Power Smoothie 28

Vegan Chocolate Power Smoothie 29

Bananarama Smoothie Recipe..30

Conclusion..31

About the Author   32

Other Books by Melinda Rolf   33

This page is intentionally left blank

Introduction

Smoothies are great snacks to perk up anyone's day. These cool concoctions can be quite refreshing during a hot day. These drinks are even made better because of the health benefits you can get from the fruits and other ingredients.

So, what can make fruit smoothies even better? You guessed it right if you said superfood. But what in the world is a superfood? It sounds a bit gimmicky. Superfood smoothies are essentially the same as other smoothies, except for the fact that they have superfoods as their main ingredient.

Of course, that's one very important difference.

What's the Deal with Superfoods?

This is practically where the controversy comes in. There are voices pro and con about the issue of superfood. Wherever you may go to find information there will be naysayers and supporters who are at each other's throats when talking about health giving foods.

Looking at from the angle of critics, the term "superfood" can be considered as a marketing gimmick. You won't hear academicians and well-respected doctors label certain foods as "super." It's not like these foods are one of a kind.

However, you should give credit to those who are in favor of superfoods. In fact, some of the supporters call it by a different name – functional food, which is actually a bit closer to the truth. These foods indeed have health-related functions.

We can definitely say that the term Superfood is a popular term for some of the popular foods that we find today. These foods somehow have a bit of bragging rights and a slight claim to the label "super." In fact, these foods are a bit unique in that they contain some of the healthiest nutrients on the planet.

Superfoods have that unique combination of being low on calories. This means that you can eat a lot of one type of superfood and you still won't go over your recommended daily caloric intake. How's that for some great weight loss?

Discover these Impressive Nutritional Perks

Now, that is only one part of the healthy combo you can get from superfoods. The other part, other than being low on calories, is the fact that they actually have a lot of nutrients. Most of them even have many anti-aging nutrients.

Needless to say, there are some marketers out there who go beyond the norm and somehow describe superfoods as some sort of magic health pill. No, these so-called superfoods are not the fountain of youth. They do not provide instant healing. They do not provide all the nutrients that you need to survive and live longer and healthier.

However, adding them to your diet kind of tips the scales in your favor where your own health is concerned. Many of these things known as superfoods actually contain a lot of antioxidants. They have the potential to help people reduce the risk of certain fatal diseases.

Really scary diseases like cancer can be dealt with if a person takes advantage of these superfoods. In fact, the American Cancer Society recommends eating foods that are rich in anti-oxidants. These foods help people get the required nutrients, while also giving them some cancer-fighting substances as well.

When you use superfoods in your smoothies, you add the same cancer-fighting nutrients into a refreshing snack or drink. Some people even use superfood smoothies as a type of meal replacement since some of them can also help lose weight.

Take note that this book supports the idea of using only natural superfoods. There are superfood products in the market today that are already processed.

You may be eating a processed form of Acai berry for instance. But that processed Acai berry fruit is really no different from other processed foods that have been stripped of their nutrients. The recipes included in this book will always make use of all natural ingredients, especially natural (not processed) superfoods.

What are Power/Superfood Ingredients?

When people talk about power foods or superfoods they often think along the lines of Acai berry, dragon fruit, deep sea seaweed, or some sort of exotic kind of fruit or food item that can you can only get from some remote part of the planet. Well, that's the initial impression. However, after going over the list of superfoods on this book, you'll find that this is more myth than fact.

In fact, many of the superfoods can actually be found and bought in a fruit stand or store. It may even surprise you to discover that some of the foods you are already eating are actually superfoods. It's also interesting that superfoods aren't limited to just fruits!

Don't think that if you go by a superfood enhanced diet that you'll be eating more fruits than you have ever done before. You'll find later in this book that certain everyday foods that are not veggies or fruits are in fact superfoods too.

What is the Special Ingredient of Superfoods?

Some people think that there must be some sort of special ingredient in superfoods that make them extra special. Sorry to burst your bubble, but it's really nothing more than phytochemicals. That's right; the big secret to why superfoods are so healthy is that they have high phytochemical content.

Phytochemicals are nutrients that are known to have the ability to help the body to fight many different types of diseases. Phytochemicals are present in many fruits, which is why some people think that superfoods are nothing more than another fruit diet in the making.

These phytochemicals actually have a lot of benefits to the human body. We have already mentioned that they fight off cancer. These nutrients also have the ability to reduce inflammation. Phytochemicals also help to strengthen the body's immune system.

In short, the phytochemicals in superfoods contribute a lot to a person's wellbeing. They make you healthier, which is a big incentive to include them in your diet. On top of that, superfoods usually taste good.

Clearing Up a Misconception

Many superfoods are actually fruits and veggies. However, some of them may not be as palatable by themselves. For instance, cocoa is a superfood. It contains a lot of flavonoids that help reduce the risk of cancer.

But have you ever tried eating some raw cocoa? Only a few people would dare do that. So, the remedy is to add some other ingredients to cocoa to make it more palatable. That is why cocoa-based superfood smoothies incorporate some sweet fruits to make the entire concoction taste really good.

The Exotic vs the Ordinary

As you will see later on, the recipes in this book don't focus on the rare superfoods that you hear about today. Other marketers have even created entire diets that are based on one or two superfoods. That's not the aim of this book.

You don't have to buy some rare fruit like noni, gogi berry, and mangosteen to get phytochemicals, vitamins, flavonoids, and probiotics. Some people will be surprised to hear that grapefruits, tomatoes, watermelons, blueberries, pomegranates, papayas, and mangoes fall into the category of superfoods.

We will not recommend any diet in this book. Instead, this book merely suggests that you include superfood smoothies in the list of food you eat each day to make your diet well-rounded and even healthier.

You should include other superfoods that may not always be included in a smoothie. Well, not all superfoods can be placed in a tall glass. Foods like garlic and soybeans won't taste good in cold glass (well, some people might like soybeans, but not everyone will love them).

The bottom line here is that you don't really have to look high and low for superfoods to include in your next smoothie recipe. Some of these superfoods may already be in your fridge! The idea is to add more of them into your meals.

Why Choose Power/Superfood Smoothies?

The big reason why people should choose to have more superfood smoothies lies in the health benefits of such refreshing beverages. Another reason why you should have them is that they are easy to prepare. You can make a power smoothie in just a couple of minutes.

Since smoothies really taste good, they are quite appealing to kids. Remember that they're not just sweet. These superfood smoothies actually taste good. They pack a lot of flavor, which means that they're not just super sweet. The smoothie recipes you'll find later in this book won't spoil your taste buds.

More Reasons to Try Superfoods

We have already mentioned that superfoods can help your body fight cancer. We have also mentioned that they can help prevent or reduce inflammation. Checking on their long term effects, superfoods have nutrients that can also help with heart disease. They have also helped some people with asthma and there are also claims that they helped people with diabetes.

There are a lot of other health benefits that people have described. Do take note that not all of them have been confirmed by science. There isn't a huge body of knowledge built around these nutrients and foods just yet.

There is evidence that these superfoods can help to detoxify the body. However, do be careful about certain types of exotic foods that are labeled as superfoods. For instance, there are certain types of seaweed that are called superfoods that can also be toxic to some people.

Many of the superfoods that are available at the store have detoxifying properties. Other than that, some of them are even known to nourish the blood. That alone can add an overall feeling of well being for the people who try them. This means that adding superfoods to your diet can also help improve your mood.

As stated earlier, there are people who use superfood smoothies to help them lose weight. It doesn't mean that the superfood ingredients will burn all the fat away. What happens actually is that the superfoods will help to naturally balance a person's appetite.

This means that you will get reduced cravings for foods that are extra sweet or extra flavorful due to additives. Since you will begin to lose your cravings for processed food (especially fast food), these superfood smoothies will help you lose weight in the long run.

There are people who have been eating superfoods for a long time and they claim that their fingernails and hair have become healthier and demonstrably stronger. There is also evidence that superfoods help with hormone imbalance and strengthen the immune system.

Since you will generally feel better about yourself (plus the added improved mood you'll have) then you will be better at handling stressful situations. Some people even use superfood smoothies as a type of convalescence food. A convalescence food is something you eat to help you recover from illness.

There are superfood smoothie recipes that are specially formulated to give people an added energy boost. This would be a healthy alternative to athletes especially those who do a lot of endurance training. Eating more superfoods will help athletes perform better in the long run.

Some people claim that since they have been eating more superfoods, they can concentrate better. They say they have gained a better mental focus. Better mental clarity is achieved as well as an improvement in their ability to concentrate.

The other good news is that many superfoods do not contain any substance that may trigger allergies. But that doesn't mean you shouldn't check if you are allergic to a certain fruit or vegetable. Most of the superfoods out there do not contain yeast or gluten so they're generally safe.

What Ingredients are the Best to Make Superfood Smoothies?

Okay, so we have already mentioned that not all superfoods will be great as part of your next smoothie. But if you're wondering what an all-garlic smoothie tastes like, then you're welcome to experiment on it. We don't really recommend it, but it's up to you if you want to spice up your next smoothie with some fresh garlic bits.

The ingredients below are some of the best ones to include in any smoothie recipe. It is not expected that you will like all of them. Some people may not be so keen with certain fruits or veggies, especially when you have to eat them raw.

Veggie smoothies may not be as popular as fruit smoothies but here's a tip: spike your superfood smoothies with some veggie bits to enhance their flavor and to add some extra healthy nutrients. That way you won't have to gulp an all veggie smoothie, but at least you're getting the best out of fruits and veggies at the same time.

In the next few pages, you'll discover some of the finest superfood smoothie ingredients.

- Avocadoes

  Avocadoes trees are native to Mexico and Central America, but they can be found just about anywhere. It is believed that they can help reduce or lower cholesterol in the blood. It is also a fact that they have high magnesium content. Magnesium is an essential nutrient to make your bones even stronger.

- Blueberries

  Blueberries are native to North America, but they can now be found in Asia and Europe as well. They look good if you add them to a smoothie. Some people consider blueberries as among the best sources of nutrients.

  The fact is that blueberries have more antioxidants compared to many superfoods that have been discovered so far. Since they have the most antioxidants, then they have more health benefits. Other than having anti-aging nutrients, blueberries are also known to help reduce a person's risk for cardiovascular diseases.

- Beans

  Not everyone is a big fan of beans even though they're readily available all over the world. There are some people who are even allergic to beans. However, despite its relative lack of popularity for some people, beans pack a lot of health benefits.

  Pinto beans, lentils, and even black beans have a lot of nutrients that will help with heart disease. It is a fact that their nutrient content can help lower blood cholesterol. They can also help stabilize a person's blood sugar levels.

  Other than the big time health benefits, these beans also have some healthy everyday uses. For instance, they can help you when experience some constipation. They also help people lose weight or avoid obesity.

- Broccoli

  The name Broccoli is Italian and this superfood has been around for more than 2,000 years. If beans are unpopular for some, what do you think about broccoli? Some kids have a terrible time with this vegetable – but it's not this veggie's fault. It's flavorless, which is its biggest downside.

  However, in spite of that lack of general appeal for a person's taste buds, broccoli is actually a very healthy veggie. It's one of the veggies that many people recommend when it comes to fighting cancer.

- Garlic

  Garlic is native to Central Asia but it has since spread worldwide. Note that we don't actually recommend garlic as the sole ingredient for your power smoothie. However, we have included it in this list so you'll remember to add a dash of garlic to your other recipes instead. You basically want garlic in your food since it is proven to help with beating certain cancers.

- Dark Chocolate

  Chocolate actually has a Mesoamerican origin. Mayans and Aztecs have been using (or rather, enjoying) chocolate centuries ago. Earlier, it was mentioned that cocoa is not a great tasting food if eaten on its own. But the good news is that cocoa is one of the ingredients for making dark chocolate. Some people think that dark chocolate is fattening – well if you eat a ton of it then it will be fattening.

But if you include it in your smoothies, then it can be a huge flavor enhancer. Other than that, it also helps you detoxify. Dark chocolate definitely belongs to the class of superfoods, which means you can have your daily dose without your conscience sneaking up on you.

Dark chocolate is a good source of phytonurtrients. It prevents the growth of unwanted blood vessels. It also has the ability to protect the DNA.

Tip: don't buy highly processed dark chocolate. We recommend the dark chocolates that don't have high cacao content. Check the labels before heading out to the cash register.

- Kiwi Fruit

The Kiwi Fruit we know today comes from northern China. However, there are other species of this fruit that come from Siberia, India, and Japan. You can find this fruit anywhere today.

You may have heard it somewhere that kiwi fruit is definitely healthy. Well, we can verify that it is true. Kiwi is one of the big stars when it comes to antioxidant rich foods. It's especially beneficial to people with heart problems. Its nutrients help reduce triglycerides. It is also found out that it can lower platelet hyperactivity.

- Honey

Honey has been used as food by humans for thousands of years. Many cultures and different countries around the world actually make use of honey. There are cave paintings in Spain that depict honey harvesters that date back to more than 8,000 years ago.

Some people may actually be allergic to honey. However, honey is definitely a staple when it comes to listing down the healthiest foods on the planet. Honey is also a good option for people who have diabetes. If you want to keep your blood-sugar levels optimal, then make sure to add some honey to your diet.

- Goji Berry (Sometimes spelled as Gogi berry)

Okay, so this is one of the rare kinds of fruits you may have seen on TV. It may not be readily available in your nearest fruit stand. In fact, you may even have to order it from some specialty store.

Goji berries are also known as wolf berries and they're originally from China. These are also known as the matrimony vine. Some countries from South America and Asia actually grow this fruit. Goji berries help improve the body's immune system, it helps protect the liver, improves eyesight, anti-aging, and improves the overall quality of the body's blood.

Of course, there are people who swear by these benefits and there are those who say it doesn't really work. Science still has to confirm whether these benefits are real or not, but that doesn't take away the fact that these berries are definitely healthy and anti-oxidant rich.

- Acai Berries

You may have heard about acai berries from the Oprah Winfrey Show or perhaps in one of Dr. Oz's shows. That's basically how Acai berries have gained popularity. Acai berries are actually one of the most nutrient foods on the planet.

No matter what you may have heard from critics, you can't take away the fact that Acai berries do have a lot of healthy nutrients. These berries actually come from the Amazon area in Brazil.

Many people say that they have slept better after adding Acai berries to their diet. The berries definitely have anti-aging properties as well. This also means that they can help boost the immune system. Some of the berry's nutrients help regulate blood cholesterol.

Some people claim that acai berries have helped them get improved vision. The nutrients in these berries definitely can help heart functions and blood circulation. There are also anti-inflammatory nutrients in these berries.

- Cacao

Cacao is rich in magnesium and iron. This means that it can help people with anemia. Its nutrients can also help women who suffer from menstrual cramps. Cacao also has a lot of manganese, which helps the body increase its amount of hemoglobin in the blood.

Cacao is also rich in zinc, which actually enhances the body's immune system. Raw cacao contains a lot of vitamin c. However, do take note that cacao does contain trans fats, so you should ease up on it and don't put too much raw or processed cacao in your smoothies.

- Maca

Maca, a fruit native to Peru, is known to increase libido. It lowers anemia levels and helps to relieve menstrual cramps too. It's a huge source of sterols. It contains vitamin E, vitamin B2, vitamin C, phosphorus, sulfur, calcium, and magnesium. Maca is also a big help to people experiencing altitude sickness.

- Spirulina

This is a type of blue-green algae, which is a food source for many ancient Mesoamericans. If you don't like the idea of eating algae then by all means you can skip on this one. You don't have to add it to your smoothie recipe.

However, take a look at its many healthy nutrients. It actually contains a lot of vitamin C, vitamin A, vitamin B complex, and vitamin E. Spirulina also contains a lot of antioxidants. It's a lot better than soy if you check out is protein building capabilities. It also helps with indigestion issues. Best of all it contains a wide array of phytonutrients, which is basically why it's considered as a superfood.

- Blue-Green Algae

The list of rare and unique superfoods is blue-green algae. You may find them sold in tablet or powder form. Again, if you're not comfortable adding them to your smoothies then don't.

Nevertheless, note that blue green algae are rich in nutrients that can lower the blood's lipid content. They're a good source of nutrients that fight off free radicals. They're also a great weight loss superfood.

- Aloe

Aloe, an Arabian Peninsula and South African native plant, is known for its ability to help the skin. Other than its cosmetic effects on the human body, aloe actually has a lot of health benefits. It can help maintain the good bacteria in the body's digestive system. It's actually a big help to people with allergies. It can help you maintain your blood sugar levels.

Aloe also contains a lot of Polysaccharides, which gives a big boost to the body's immune system. It contains a lot of nutrients that enables the body to detoxify. It also helps prevent fungus infections.

These are only some of the ingredients that you can include in your power smoothie recipes. You'll like some of them, but we don't expect that you will like all of them. Just choose the superfoods that appeal to you. Remember that you can always include a pinch or two of some new superfood ingredients to add to your recipe from time to time.

Power Smoothie Recipes to Boost Your Health

The following are some of our recommended power smoothie or superfood smoothies that will help give you a good health boost. You can pick out some of your favorites too if you want. Remember that you can also alter the recipes and tweak them in terms of taste.

You can also create your own power smoothie recipes too. You can use some of the recipes as a template and just mix and match ingredients along the way. The important thing is to include superfoods in your diet. If you're ready to learn how to prepare the finest smoothies, simply flip the page.

Citrus Aloe Vera Smoothie Recipe

This is a refreshing smoothie that aids in detoxifying your body. The combination of citrus fruits and aloe vera is perfect for eliminating toxins. Other than being ideal for detoxification, aloe is also good for your heart and overall cardiovascular health.

Ingredients:

- 1/2 piece of medium-sized lime, (peeled with seeds removed)
- 1/2 piece of avocado
- 1 tablespoon of coconut oil
- 1/2 piece of medium-sized lemon, (peeled with seeds removed)
- 1 cup of water
- A dash of Celtic sea salt
- 1 piece of medium-sized aloe vera leaf
- 1 tablespoon honey

Optional Ingredients:

- 1 tablespoon of chia or flax seeds
- 1 cup of green leaves like spinach, kale, etc.
- 1 piece of kiwi, peeled
- Other healthy fruits and vegetables that are readily available in your pantry

Instructions:

Mix all the ingredients in a high-speed blender for 30 seconds. In case your blender isn't a high speed model, you should blend all the ingredients minus the coconut oil. Doing this will help to prevent the ingredients from forming clumps; which makes it hard for your machine to process all the ingredients.

Once all the ingredients have been blended, you can drizzle the smoothie with the coconut oil on top and serve. You can even blend the oil in for 3 to 5 seconds before serving.

Coconut + Cranberry Power Smoothie

The coconut is considered as the tree of life. Coconuts are actually one of the healthiest foods on the planet. They help improve digestion, they are great for the brain, and they can help increase thyroid production. Cranberries on the other hand are rich in antioxidants, which help the body fight cancer.

Ingredients:

- ¾ cup fresh orange juice
- 1 cup ice cubes
- 2 frozen bananas
- 1 cup cultured coconut yogurt
- 1 cup fresh cranberries
- 1 teaspoon vanilla extract
- A pinch of salt

Instructions:

Place all the ingredients in a blender. Blend everything until creamy. Pour the contents in a glass.

Pistachio Superfood Smoothie

Pistachios are one of the best tasting nuts on the planet. They are good for the heart and they can also help people with diabetes. They can also help improve eye health and strengthen the nervous system. It's time to start shelling those pistachios since you're making a nice smoothie out of them.

Ingredients:

- 4 regular sized dates
- 1 cup pistachio cream
- Maca powder
- ½ cup avocado oil
- ¼ cup rolled oats
- ⅛ teaspoon vanilla
- 5 ice cubes
- ½ banana
- ¾ cup spinach (chopped)
- ¼ cup organic pistachios
- ¼ cup coconut whip

Instructions:

Place all ingredients inside your blender.
Blend until everything gets incorporated and mixed evenly.
Pour the mixture in a tall glass or pitcher. Serve cold.

The Energizer Smoothie

Do you feel weak right in the middle of a working day? Pick yourself up and get that added strength boost with this power smoothie. It provides the health benefits of coconuts and honey. Wheatgrass gives your body a big boost of energy, while honey is good for the digestive tract.

Ingredients:

- 1 cup coconut water
- 1 tablespoon of honey
- 1/2 cup mango
- 1 teaspoon wheatgrass powder
- 1/2 cup kale
- 1 teaspoon maca
- 2 tablespoons goji berries
- 1 teaspoon coconut oil
- 1 tablespoon coconut flakes
- 1/2 avocado
- 1/2 cup spinach
- 1/3 cup Greek yogurt
- 2 tablespoons dried cranberries

Instructions:

Place all the ingredients inside your blender.
Blend for half a minute.
Place contents in your smoothie glass.
Enjoy and be reinvigorated.

Spirulina Power Smoothie

This smoothie will help you get a taste of spirulina. Even if you don't like the idea of gulping down some algae, this smoothie may help get you that needed acquired taste for something really healthy. It has high amounts of calcium, which is good for the teeth. It's also rich in vitamins which help the body fight diseases.

Ingredients:

- 1 tablespoon of spirulina
- 1 cup spinach leaves
- 1 green apple (cored)
- Honey
- 1 1/2 cups apple juice
- 1 cucumber (peeled and sliced)

Instructions:

Place all these ingredients in a blender.
Blend everything for 20 to 30 seconds or until you get an even consistency.
Place contents in a glass. Enjoy.

Vegan Chocolate Power Smoothie

Chocolate tastes good, right? Adding vegetables to chocolate makes it even healthier. Check out what chocolate and veggies taste like. The nutrients contained in chocolate can help improve blood pressure and reduce heart attack. It can also help increase insulin sensitivity.

Ingredients:

- 1 cup almond milk
- 2 tablespoons cacao powder
- 1 tablespoon Maca
- 1 tablespoon chia seeds
- 1 fresh banana
- A few dates
- 1 cup blueberries

Instructions:

Blend all ingredients in high setting.
Blend until you get a creamy, even consistency.
Pour contents in your smoothie glass.
Enjoy while it's fresh.

Bananarama Smoothie Recipe

You will enjoy all the healthy benefits of bananas with this super smoothie since as the main ingredient. Combined with other healthy foods, you will definitely enjoy this very nutritious recipe. Eating bananas can help you overcome depression and it's also good for your digestive tract.

Ingredients:

- 1 piece of banana, frozen or fresh
- 2 tablespoons of Greek yogurt
- 1 1/2 cups of almond milk, homemade is better
- 1/2 cup of strawberries, frozen or fresh
- 1 tablespoon of chia seed gel or chia seeds
- 1 cup of spinach
- 1 teaspoon of bee pollen
- 1/2 cup of mango chunks, frozen or fresh
- 1 tablespoon of coconut oil

Optional Ingredients:

- 1 tablespoon of hemp seeds
- honey
- 1 tablespoon of Gelatin or any protein powder of your preference
- 1 cup of kale

Instructions:

Put everything your blender.
Blend all ingredients for 30 seconds or until the texture becomes smooth and consistent.

You have the option to add the coconut oil later, in case your blender is having a hard time mixing everything up.
You can add it once the smoothie finally has the right consistency.
Drizzle it on top and blend it before serving.
This will prevent the ingredients from forming into clumps.

Conclusion

Superfood smoothies can add a huge boost of healthy nutrients to anyone's diet. You can also use them as meal replacements to help you lose weight. Remember that you can always include other superfoods in the sample recipes provided in this book.

Have fun experimenting on different flavors. Once again, thank you for getting this book. Hopefully, the information here helped you in your quest for better health.

About the Author

Melinda is a superfood junkie and mom of three

Now she has decided to share some of her tips and recipes with you. She hopes you will enjoy them as much as she and her family do

Melinda is also an avid cook and soap maker has made hundreds of soaps and sells them at many of her local flea markets, festivals, and other local and regional events.

She has written a book on the subject which is also available at Amazon.

Melinda lives with her husband, 3 children 2 dogs, a cat, and a yellow bellied turtle in Swanville, Maine

If you have enjoyed this book, please leave me a nice review at Amazon, I really appreciate it. Melinda

Other Books by Melinda Rolf

Prep Freeze Serve
Prep Freeze Serve Chicken
Crockpot Recipes
African Black Soap
How to Make Natural Handmade Soap
Loom Jewelry for Beginners
The Raw Deal: The Benefits of a Raw Food Diet

Available at Amazon